Acknowledgements

We would like to acknowledge the support of the Research & Development Directorate of the NHSE London Regional Office and, in particular, of David Evans, Implementation Facilitator.

Several colleagues from the King's Fund and elsewhere provided helpful and constructive comments on the draft final report, and we are most grateful to them.

We would also like to thank all of the project team members who led the work in their health authorities, and who made this evaluation possible through their enthusiasm and commitment. Finally, we thank their colleagues in the projects for taking the time to respond to our questions.

*They know, they **know** the knowledge. We often start from the assumption that people need to be told all this stuff, that they need to have it reinforced. But it isn't about that. It isn't about more guidelines; it's about getting that behaviour changed.*

Project lead

Getting better with evidence

Experiences of putting evidence into practice

Lesley Wye (née Smith)

John McClenahan

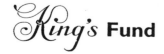

Published by
King's Fund Publishing
11–13 Cavendish Square
London W1G 0AN

© King's Fund 2000

First published 2000

ISBN 1 85717 420 8

A CIP catalogue record for this book is available from the British Library

Available from:

King's Fund Bookshop
11–13 Cavendish Square
London
W1G 0AN

Tel: 020 7307 2591
Fax: 020 7307 2801

Printed and bound in Great Britain

Contents

Executive Summary

Putting evidence into practice is a lengthy, complicated process. Despite a growing body of literature on effective strategies, many health professionals continue to struggle.

The former North Thames (now London Region) Research & Development Directorate made their contribution to this field with the *Purchaser-Led Implementation Projects Programme*. In 1995, each of the region's 14 health authorities were asked to submit a bid for £50,000 to put one or more pieces of 'robust' evidence into practice. Seventeen projects from 15 project teams were funded for 18 months.

The King's Fund was asked to establish the effectiveness of different approaches. Specifically, we were to look at objectives and planned outcomes, barriers and how the approaches used could be generalised.

Using mainly qualitative methods over almost three years, we found that four areas were crucial. With these things in place, success seems more likely (but not guaranteed):

- resources – of time, money and skills – need to be sufficient
- the proposed change needs to offer benefits of interest to frontline staff
- enough of the right people (everyone affected by the change, and in particular senior clinical leaders) need to be on board early enough
- the approach needs to be interactive and relate research clearly to current practice.

We also found that other valuable outcomes usually occurred before a change in clinical practice or demonstrable improvements in patient care. The four stages of project development are shown in the following diagram.

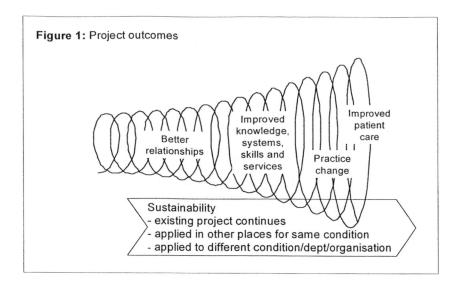

Figure 1: Project outcomes

Fifteen of the 17 project teams established **better relationships** between organisations/departments and/or between members of clinical teams.

Eleven of the 17 projects continue to **improve knowledge, systems, services and skills**; one stopped before achieving this. Without these four elements in place, a change in practitioners' behaviour cannot be supported or sustained.

Three of the 17 projects brought about a systematic **change in clinical practice**. Local health professionals from two of the three felt that behavioural change was now thoroughly embedded into routine practice. Local health professionals from two of the three mentioned that **improved patient care** was also being achieved.

Key lessons from project teams were:

- expect to take several *years*, not 18 months, to change clinical behaviour
- while getting high quality *evidence* takes a rigorous, and highly pre-planned approach, successful *implementation* requires pragmatism and flexibility
- start small and build incrementally
- use what is already there (such as regular team meetings, educational events, communication forums, audit processes) and build on previous work
- target enthusiasts first.

Project summary table

Project type	Topic	Intervention
Cardiac/stroke projects		
Barking & Havering	Secondary prevention of CHD	Guidelines 1:1 feedback from audit to practice teams Prompts Formal presentations Systematic clinics Opinion leaders
Brent & Harrow	Open-access non-invasive cardiac diagnostic services	Open-access services (echo, ECG, etc.) Training session w/GPs only
East London & the City	Cardiac intervention	Formal presentation 5 multi-disc training workshops 1 standalone computer on ward
Hertfordshire	Nurse-led anti-coagulation clinics	Guidelines Face to face, small group training (14 sessions in 3 months) Led by senior cons Nurse-led clinics Computer dosing package
Kensington, Chelsea & Westminister	Open-access echocardiography	Guidelines Open-access echo service Practice meetings on service expectations
South Essex	Hypertension in elderly people	Guidelines 7 seminars to GPs and practice nurses Incentives
H pylori		
Camden & Islington	h pylori & dyspepsia	Guidelines Self-audit pack for GP practices Incentives Distance learning pack
Hillingdon	h pylori	Guidelines Formal presentations 3 informal question and answer sessions w/GPs Ad hoc meetings w/GPs Incentives Serology service
Leg ulcers		
East London & the City	Leg ulcers	Guidelines Led by senior nurse specialist Monthly face to face training while patient in consultation 2 nurse-led clinics
Hillingdon	Leg ulcers	Guidelines Formal presentations 3 ½ day training sessions for all district nurses and ¼ practice nurses Increased access to prescription ortho wool and Doppler ultrasound
Diabetes		
Barnet	Diabetes retinopathy	Guidelines 2 clinics Opinion leaders
Ealing, Hounslow & Hammersmith	Diabetes register	Workshops on data collection Opinion leader Practice visits on data collection Incentives Feedback of data collection

Internal evaluation	Outcome
Cardiac/stroke projects	
Patient note audit	Audit + prompt + clinic = **practice change** (30–32%) Audit alone = modest level of practice change in prescribing (17%) Audit + prompt = modest level of practice change (15–16%)
Audit on behavioural intentions, waiting times, costs, number of patients treated in primary vs secondary care	Very modest change in practice (7% of patients on effective treatments)
Independent, qualitative evaluation	Limited improvement in nurses' interest in computing
Patient outcomes (stroke admissions)	**Embedded practice change**
Patient note audit (not available to external evaluators) Qualitative evaluation on best practice	Better relationships between organisations Increased GP knowledge Extent of practice change not known
Patient note audit	Better relationships between organisations Increased GP knowledge No change in practice
H pylori	
Patient note audit PACT data	Better relationships between organisations Increased GP knowledge Patient note data = 291+ patients on treatment PACT data = no change
Referrals to serology service PACT data	Better relationships between organisations Referrals to serology service at expected level PACT data = significant decrease in number of items prescribed
Leg ulcers	
Negligible	**Practice change** – possibly not embedded yet
Patient note data collected by district nurses on use of bandaging and Doppler ultrasound Qualitative questionnaire on knowledge and attitudes	Better relationships between organisations Increased use of Doppler (up from 66% to 95%)
Diabetes	
Pending	Better relationships between organisations Extent of practice change not known
Data on numbers of newly recorded patients, annual reviews, investigations	Better relationships between organisations 17% more diabetic patients found in pilot practices Extent of practice change not known

Project summary table (continued)

Project type	Topic	Intervention
Other primary care topics		
Barnet	Low back pain	Guidelines 3 problem-based workshops Opinion leader Physio service re-configuration
Enfield & Haringey	GP learning sets	2 GP only and 2 GP + practice nurse or pharmacist groups Discussions on evidence for various topics Incentives
Redbridge & Waltham Forest	Diabetes, hypertension, asthma	Guidelines Formal presentations Locality workshops Practice-based meetings, changes needed to implement guidelines
Other secondary care topics		
Brent & Harrow	A&E protocols	Guidelines (protocols) for 24 minor and 11 major conditions Protocol necessary for every patient presenting as no other documentation available Led by senior cons
North Essex	Cancer services	Guidelines Guidelines on web site One to one meetings to raise awareness

Internal evaluation	Outcome
Other primary care topics	
Audit of inappropriate referrals	Better relationships between organisations Audit showed inappropriate referrals went down and back up again
Patient note audit on some topics (not available to external evaluators)	Better relationships between GPs No evidence of practice change
Various types of patient note audit (not available to external evaluators)	Better relationships between organisations and clinical teams Better admin systems Extent of practice change not known
Other secondary care topics	
Data on protocol usage available to external evaluators Data on appropriateness of selection and adherence to standards (not available)	**Embedded practice change**
Audit on referral times and type	Better relationships between doctors No evidence of practice change

1. Introduction

1.1 The regional programme

There have been several programmes funded in the past decade that explore the gap between producing evidence and putting that evidence into practice.[1, 2, 3, 4] In 1995, the former North Thames Research & Development Directorate set up their contribution by funding 15 project teams to carry out 17 projects.

They invited all of the 14 former North Thames health authorities to submit one or more proposals to implement a piece of 'robust' evidence. Each health authority received £50,000 and the projects were funded for 18 months.

Most (officially) started with the appointment of a project worker in 1997 and funding continued to 1998. The programme was health authority based and a high proportion of the projects focused on improvements in primary care (eight), while the rest were in secondary care (four), at the interface between primary and secondary care (three), or in community care (two). (See project summary on preceding pages.)

Of the 15 teams, eight were based in health authorities, four in secondary care, one in the local Multidisciplinary Audit Advisory Group (MAAG), one in a community trust and one team ran jointly between the health authority and a secondary care provider.

1.2 The external evaluation

The regional brief to the King's Fund

We were asked to establish the effectiveness of the projects' different approaches. Specifically, we were to look at:

- outcomes and to what extent they had been achieved
- barriers identified and overcome
- generalisability of approach in terms of topic and location.

We took this one step further and looked at factors that helped clinicians to integrate research evidence into daily practice in a sustainable way. (For a full account, please see the report, including appendices, which will be available for download from the King's Fund (www.kingsfund.org.uk/Publishing/html/publications_free_download.cfm) and/or North Thames web sites.)

1.3 Evaluation design

We selected a developmental evaluation model for four main reasons.

1. It is especially helpful when the item for evaluation changes during the study period and/or is poorly defined.
2. It encourages participants to set their own objectives, reflect on what they have learned and change course as necessary.
3. It allows for changes in the evaluation methodology as and when needed.
4. It allowed us to move from detached observation to action research.[5]

1.4 Constructing a framework for analysis

In April 1997 we held a workshop to define 'success', to which we invited 15 professionals with experience in implementation. The eight who were able to attend were a medical director, a GP, a voluntary organisation director, a health authority chief executive, a senior nursing lecturer, an academic, a representative from the Centre for Reviews and Dissemination (CRD) and the implementation facilitator for North Thames R&D.

They defined 'success' as either:

- a project that meets all of its objectives OR
- a project that does not fully meet its objectives, but in which individuals and the organisation analyse why and learn from it.

They also identified a set of nine elements of success against which the projects could be assessed.[6] The elements were:

- undertaking **groundwork** thoroughly

- choosing a good **leader**

- involving **users** (defined as local professionals as well as patients)

- creating the right **environment** within the organisation

- **facilitating the change** before meeting resistance

- **overcoming barriers** after meeting resistance

- **avoiding hindrances** where possible

- incorporating **evaluation**

- encouraging **sustainability**

1.5 Sources of data on the projects

By the end of the evaluation (autumn 1999) we had several sources of data.

- *Workshop notes.* We held three series of workshops, to which all of the project teams were invited. The first focused on objectives and evaluation. The second was on evidence, barriers to implementation and strategies for overcoming them. The third looked at sustainability once North Thames funding ended.

- *Telephone surveys.* We conducted two qualitative telephone surveys with three to six local health professionals (who were not members of the project teams). This provided external confirmation of impressions we received during the workshops.

- *Final and interim reports.* Eleven of the teams wrote a chapter for a forthcoming book edited by David Evans and Andrew Haines,[7] which were submitted instead of a final report. Four other teams wrote final reports.

- *Self-assessment questionnaires.* At least one member, and sometimes two, completed a questionnaire on strengths, weaknesses and successes of their project.

2. Analysis

2.1 Difficulties in carrying out an evaluation of this nature

Mutability of the projects

These projects were constantly evolving, so evaluation could only provide a snapshot in time. What can look initially very promising can falter and stall a few months later. For example, at our last workshop sustainability looked good for a primary care project. Five months later, two members of the team have left or are leaving, making its future unclear.

Definitions of 'success'

The external expert group defined success in two ways: meeting objectives and/or learning from experience. In reality, this created problems. Firstly, overly ambitious original objectives had to be refined in the face of what was achievable. Due to this, success was secured against these more feasible objectives. Secondly, lessons could be learned in all cases, meaning that even ineffectual projects could be 'successful'.

Lack of data measuring clinical change according to the evidence

Four of the project teams were able to collect robust data from the practitioners involved, and three of these were able to pass that data on to us. By 'robust' data we mean that these teams directly measured how practitioners' behaviour changed before and after their interventions, and whether patients were now receiving more effective and appropriate treatments.

Other projects collected data that did not show this causal link. One collected a small quantity of data (<55 patients), which were not sufficient.

Some teams collected *process* data (e.g. number of practitioners attending an event), which are useful in gauging interest but say little about the degree of practice change.

Others gathered *proxy* data, which, whilst an indicator of trends, is not a direct measurement. These proxy data often took the form of information on service and equipment usage (e.g. Doppler ultrasounds, open-access echocardiography, numbers of referrals). These may indicate that practitioners made some changes in their behaviour (e.g. they used a piece of equipment more), but we do not know if they followed up diagnoses appropriately or if they were using the equipment correctly, according to guidelines.

PACT prescription data were another common source of proxy data. These may indicate a change in trends, but again do not directly measure the extent of change. For example, one project team collected both PACT data and practice data. PACT data indicated no change in overall prescribing rates, but patient notes showed that nearly 300 new patients had been prescribed more effective treatments.

Without robust data, we have had to rely on self-reports by the project teams and the frontline staff expected to make the changes. This can be misleading. For example, practitioners in one project said they were now treating elderly people with hypertension at lower blood pressure levels. While genuinely believing that they were now acting in line with the evidence and that their clinical behaviour was different, data collected in 16 practices for over 5000 patients showed that no significant change had occurred.

We began our analysis with the above restrictions. However, we did have robust patient-related data from three projects: one shows no or limited change; one shows varying levels of change depending on the intervention; and one shows modest levels of change. We also had a large body of qualitative data from different sources.

2.2 Outcomes analysis

Using information from the project teams (workshop notes and reports) and local professionals (two surveys), we listed all of the perceived outcomes. We also gained an understanding of the level of importance attached to them by the frequency and emphasis by which they were mentioned.

We devised a wheel based on the top 12 items. Each item was defined and we rated each project's progress as none, low, medium or high. These ratings were on the basis of information we had as of the last contact with the projects.

Figure 2: Did it make a difference?

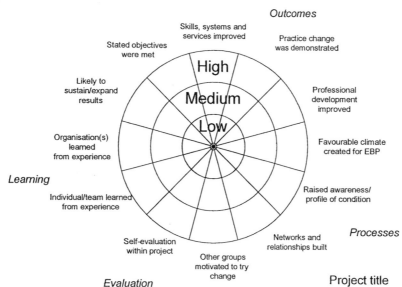

With the wheel, we now had a picture for each project. The ones that seemed to have greatest success had most segments shaded on the diagram. We were able to classify projects by level of progress but still did not know what factors had led to that progress.

2.3 Process analysis

We then selected the wheels for the projects that had made the most progress. We applied the broad themes identified by the external expert group in a case study approach. We also noted anything that surprised or refuted our own beliefs. After identifying key factors that helped progress for each, we summarised them. We now had a preliminary list.

Using the same case study approach, we then looked at the:

- three projects that had made the least progress
- three projects with data that directly measured a change in clinical behaviour
- remaining eight projects.

We now had a list of nine items that helped projects make progress. Several of our items could be grouped together. With this revised, shorter list, we went back to all of the projects and re-analysed to see if our findings were sound.

3. Four key factors seem to be essential

We found four factors that are key to putting evidence into practice.

- Resources – of time, money and skills – need to be sufficient.
- The proposed change needs to offer benefits of interest to frontline staff.
- Enough of the right people (everyone affected by the change, and in particular senior clinical leaders) need to be on board early enough.
- The approach needs to be interactive and relate research clearly to current practice.

3.1 Resources need to be sufficient

Which resources and who needs them?

Adequate money, skills and time were essential. Without initial funding from North Thames, many of these projects would not have been started.

By skills, we mean both applied (computing and auditing) and interpersonal (change management and communication). In addition, two groups of people needed these resources – those who made the change (frontline staff) and those who managed the change (project teams).

Time was the resource in shortest supply. A continuing frustration was that funding was only for 18 months:

> It's the same problem with all evidence-based projects. They take a long time to set up and the money runs out just when it's about to take off and you can't show any benefits yet.

Ideally, project teams could use North Thames funding to develop something that could carry on without further money:

Rather than just use extra money to parachute in, try to use the money to build capacity for the training and development of staff. Once you have a clinic in there, if you've re-organised the systems then when the money goes away, the system's still in place. In diabetes we know that we need to do this, but the district nurses are so overloaded with patients that they don't have the time. You need development money and time.

Time is scarce for everyone, but practitioners were willing to make the time – if the benefits were of sufficient value.

3.2 The proposed change needs to offer benefits of real interest to staff who have to change

What benefits do staff want?

Making change means considerable extra work for frontline practitioners. Although staff were grateful (and often surprised) to receive thanks or recognition, that alone was not sufficient to get them to change their behaviour.

The benefits that most motivated staff were:

- savings in time
- savings in money
- improved patient care
- professional development (for nurses).

Interestingly, professional development was not reported as motivating doctors or managers.

Project teams that could capitalise on the operational concerns of frontline staff found progress easier:

Practices were much more likely to take up an offer of support in introducing a guideline when it related to one of their own priority areas. In our case this resulted in the favourable reaction to the hypertension guidelines and the generally negative response to the antibiotic prescribing guidelines, which was perceived to be 'outside imposition'.

Motivation was poor if only one group benefited when many others had to put in the work. However if more than one type of benefit was available for more than one group, then progress was easier.

For example, one project was unusual in that it led to an all round win/win situation:

Everyone has won. It's an improved service for the patient. It's good employment for two nurses ... Junior doctors benefit. There are savings in out-patients, so the trust benefits. And the nurses have relieved the consultants of hours of work [the consultants found] dull and repetitive.

3.3 Enough of the right people need to be on board early enough

Who are the right people?

Everyone affected by the change

A few of the project teams accurately identified and included all potential stakeholders from the beginning:

[One of its strengths is] it involved a broad spectrum of professionals – Public Health, gastroenterologists, health authority advisors, GPs.

Some project teams had too narrow a focus or identified key professionals too late:

They got the right people in the same room at the end, but not enough in the beginning. GPs were in the dark and the consultants were not really happy.

A few did not clarify whom to include since they were not sure what they wanted to do:

It needed a much clearer set of objectives as consultants were not involved from the beginning. No one seemed to know what to do, least of all X [project worker].

Many project teams were not based inside their target organisations and did not know how those organisations worked:

> *The project was primarily aimed at GPs because of our assumption that GPs initiate treatment for hypertension ... With hindsight we should have made a much greater effort to involve practice nurses as well as GPs. Practice nurses have become increasingly responsible for the screening and management of hypertension in the elderly.*

Several project teams mentioned that it would have been easier to locate the project team appropriately if they had thought about it earlier and more systematically:

> *With hindsight, we consider that a systematic assessment of the networks within primary care should have been made before deciding on the location of the project [team].*

The senior clinical leader

If the senior clinical leader was indifferent (at best), sceptical, or even hostile (at worst), then progress was difficult.

One team was publicly challenged by a senior consultant opposed to the project. The project worker wrote:

> *This intense challenge to the legitimacy of the project had quite a profound effect on the subsequent interest and enthusiasm shown by the hospital staff.*

Why do they not want to get on board?

Sometimes, staff do not want to take part because there are no benefits for them, as discussed earlier. The proposed change may also be perceived as shifting the balance of power:

> *This concern related to the possibility of juniors usurping the role of seniors ('if juniors can get advice from a machine, will they bypass their seniors?'). It also related to clinicians' worries that 'nurses would tell doctors how to do their job.'*

3.4 The approach needs to be interactive and relate research to current practice

What approaches do teams usually use?

Faced with changing the clinical behaviour of large numbers of professionals, most project teams organised large workshops or presentations. Local practitioners then knew about the project, but few subsequently changed their clinical behaviour:

> *The dissemination of information is difficult. We did it through lectures. But lots of GPs take things into their own hands and prescribe what they want anyway.*

Which approach is more likely to lead to success?

To get clinical behavioural change, a more resource-intensive approach was required. Project teams:

- used a non-threatening, face to face approach
- met one on one or in small groups (e.g. practice or clinical team)
- related the ideal (research evidence) to current practice
- planned for ways to improve practice
- repeatedly went back to identify and overcome practical difficulties as they arose.

For example, in one project a clinical nurse specialist visited once a month and worked directly with nurses while patients were in consultation. When asked if the project had made any difference to her clinical practice, one nurse said:

> *Definitely. Having her [the clinical nurse specialist] there to discuss different things helps. When you are seeing seven leg ulcers in a row, it leads to better practice. We are using the leg ulcer care programme [guidelines] lots.*

What happens if the approach is not right

If project teams had managed the other three areas well enough, but had difficulties in this area, they were still likely to generate something:

The only difference [the project has made] is that it has flagged up awareness.

In a few cases, sustained clinical practice change did occur, despite the lack of an interactive approach. This was amongst those practitioners who had the enthusiasm, resources and skills to carry on by themselves:

The willingness of practice members to engage in it [made the project possible]. Their maturity ... We discovered from the audit cycle we were very high on smoking but not on aspirin ... when we reaudited, we saw some improvement but not much. The practice nurse said we need a proper clinic for systematic monitoring ... We now need to re-audit. The practice didn't get any funding for this.

4. Successive outcomes in implementing change

4.1 Better relationships

The first outcome of substantial value was an improvement in relationships. At least one project team member or local health professional from 15 of the 17 projects commented that better relationships had been established.

This occurred between people from different professions and/or between organisations:

> *It's forged wonderful relationships between the health authority, the practices and the physiotherapists who are practice based.*

For some of the project teams, this improvement in relationships was the real endpoint to their work:

> *After all isn't better relationships really what all this is about?*

Some project teams found that, despite patchy progress in changing clinical behaviour, these relationships were very valuable because of current priorities:

> *One of the byproducts has been the relationships between the GPs and Public Health ... The new clinical governance leads already are seeing the benefit because GPs are more primed than they were before.*

4.2 Knowledge, skills, systems and services

The second outcome is more complex as it involves four elements. Project teams often found that their relationships with others improved while working towards this outcome.

In terms of **knowledge**, project teams and frontline staff needed to clarify:

- what staff *should be* doing (according to the evidence)
- what they *are* doing
- how to bridge the gap between the two.

We need a step in the middle – how to assess the evidence for their own practice. GPs need more training in appraising the evidence and seeing how it applies to their own practice.

In looking at **skills**, because computing and auditing skills were in such short supply, all but one project team carried out audits themselves:

... the lack of computer skills was a further barrier to implementation in many practices. Most did not have 'in house' the skills to audit current practice by computer query.

There was a clear lack of consistency and quality of data entry within and across practices. For example, raised blood pressure can have at least five different Read codes, and in many practices, all had been used!

The **services** required were different for every project. Examples included serology testing, physiotherapy redistribution, diabetes retinopathy clinics, open-access non-invasive cardiac diagnostic services, nurse-led anti-coagulation clinics and leg ulcer clinics. Not every project team needed to set up or re-configure services, but they all had to consider if current provision could support the proposed change:

Invest more time in developing and standardising access to relevant diagnostic testing across the health authority. (A lot of hard work in educating and persuading people to change what they are doing can be undermined by practical limitations such as inequality of access to necessary services.)

Exploring how to make local **systems** work in favour of the change was not straightforward. Project teams often forgot about the ways things currently work, which can prevent change happening:

An administrative system [made this possible] – nothing technical or clever. Just getting things organised ... It's not a knowledge gap with practitioners. They know it all. But they have problems in how to organise it ... We had a first audit and then a second and nothing had changed. So then we re-organised things and it improved.

Nearly three years on, 11 projects are still working towards this series of outcomes and one has stopped before reaching them.

4.3 Practice change

Once the previously mentioned outcomes are achieved, a change in practitioners' behaviour occurs whereby they act systematically (not partially or haphazardly) according to the evidence. Three of the projects were successful in this:

The feel is ongoing, we can't stop now ... We have a culture of evidence-based medicine in the department now. It's very dynamic. We couldn't go back to the way we were before.

Of the three projects that achieved this, only two were considered by local health professionals to be embedded.

It's an enormous achievement to get change in this climate and [the project lead] has done it ... Possibly it's not sufficiently embedded yet. There is still lots of development work to happen ... It needs a couple of years' more push.

For those two that did become embedded, teams accomplished this by making it impossible to work as they did before. For example, one team set up a system so that a nurse or SHO prints out the appropriate protocol from a computer for every patient that comes in. In part, protocol usage is high because:

You have to use them. There is nothing else to write on.

4.4 Improved patient care

If the evidence is correct, once practice changes systematically and routinely then patients benefit from improved quality of care:

The results are better. There are not so many patients with horrible ongoing ulcers as before. Patients are very satisfied.

4.5 Sustainability

We defined sustainability in three ways:

- the current project continues after North Thames funding finished
- the model of the project has been applied elsewhere, in the same context
- the model of the project has been applied to other conditions or in other departments/organisations.

Projects did not have to reach the stage of improved patient care to show signs of sustainability: ten of the 17 projects are still going in some form; one has been applied elsewhere for the same condition; four have been applied to other conditions, departments or organisations. Two have stopped.

5. Conclusions

5.1 A spiral model of change

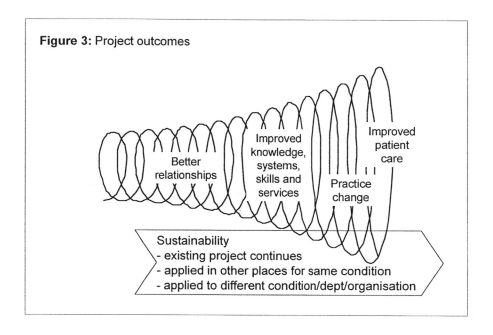

Figure 3: Project outcomes

Better relationships

Improved knowledge, systems, skills and services

Practice change

Improved patient care

Sustainability
- existing project continues
- applied in other places for same condition
- applied to different condition/dept/organisation

Progress is not linear

We have illustrated changing clinical behaviour as a sideways spiral. Project teams emphasised that practice change does not come about by developing pre-specified and fixed objectives, by setting out plans for their realisation and methodically ticking them off as completed (like scaling a ladder):

> *In this kind of work, objectives are like moving targets.*

Instead, project teams found their experience to be a case of 'three steps forward and two steps back'. If a mistake was severe enough, progress slipped quite far back. For example, one team was working towards guidelines that many GPs did not think were feasible:

> *My colleagues give me flak because they are gold standard rather than what could be done practically. It's turning GPs away rather than involving them.*

This team worked hard to re-engage GPs and later guidelines were much more practical. One year later, some local professionals query guidelines coming from any other source.

The spiral reflects the up and down, emotional nature of this work:

> *This can be very disheartening work because you are bringing in your skills but not new resources and 'carrots'. It's a lot of saying 'let's do this and maybe you'll get this', when quite often you don't have control over the 'maybe'. It can be discouraging.*

The scope of work amplifies over time

A spiral that starts small and grows bigger also mirrors how the projects 'amplified'. Most teams involved the obvious professionals first, but that circle widened to encompass those from other professions and organisations:

> *Start small and then grow sideways. It's easier in places like X, which is a small district with only one provider.*

The scope of the change also grew as teams resolved a range of difficulties:

> *It is clear that any policy to encourage the adoption of effective clinical care needs to take a wide view so that a whole range of potential organisational, financial and professional barriers are taken into account.*

Implementation is the real work: guidelines are not enough

In general, project teams agreed:

> *Guidelines on their own do nothing. Patients come in with back pain and the GP shunts them off to the physiotherapist. This is more likely than the GP looking at the guideline.*

Although difficult enough, it was easier for some project teams to focus on developing guidelines:

> *If 'guidelines' is in the project title, then simply getting guidelines produced is a good enough outcome.*

The much harder task of implementing was sometimes under-prioritised:

With hindsight, we feel that we may have succumbed to the temptation to produce an impressive document at the expense of the main objective, changing practice.

5.2 Advice to others from the project teams

Key messages from the project teams to others undertaking similar work were:[6, 8]

- Expect to take several years, not 18 months, to change clinical behaviour:

Everything takes three times long as you expect.

We have found that continuous effort is required to embed the use of guidelines into everyday practice, and we would suggest that this is a process which is best considered in a timeframe of years rather than months.

It takes at least five years.

- Be flexible and tailor your approach:

We came to realise as the project evolved that greater flexibility was a virtue, and would be a strength rather than a weakness. It is in this respect that the contrast between the rigorous, inflexible approach which gives rise to the highest quality research evidence and the flexible, pragmatic approach necessary for research implementation is most marked.

GPs are individuals whose interests, priorities, motivations and needs all differ. An attempt to engage them must recognise and adapt to these differences.

- Start small and build incrementally:

Concentrate on a small number of topics initially; expand only when you have gained experience (yourself), and the confidence of others.

We came to appreciate the importance of piloting ... with a small number of participating practices because it enabled us to iron out the problems which came to light ... before rolling out to a large number of practices.

- Use what is already there (such as regular team meetings, educational events, communication forums, audit processes) and build on previous work:

  Start from where local work is already happening.

  Use an educational approach and plug into credible existing frameworks.

  The project was part of a bigger initiative which was itself one component of a wider development agenda in the Trust.

- Target enthusiasts first:

  If audit is to be used, pilot it with practices with a keen interest in audit rather than a high need group.

  [We] also found it effective to focus attention on the least unenthusiastic member of each team, looking for (and often achieving), a 'knock on' effect to their colleagues.

5.3 Did the projects make a difference?

Even those projects that made very limited progress in changing practice still benefited someone. For example, one of the otherwise least successful projects resulted in:

... some of the nursing staff [developing] their own ways of managing their discomfort with new technology. An 'informal economy' of equipping and training ward nurses had developed ... Training was provided by one nurse who was experienced in computing and knowledgeable about programs.

Changing practice is a lengthy, complicated process. Regardless of the degree of progress made, the project teams should be commended for their hard work and commitment. They all made a difference.

References

1. Dopson SE and Gabbay J. *Getting Research into Practice and Purchasing: Issues and Lessons from the Four Counties.* Commissioned by Anglia & Oxford Region. Wessex Institute of Public Health Medicine & Templeton College, 1995.

2. Dunning M *et al. Experience, Evidence and Everyday Practice.* London: King's Fund, 1999.

3. Humphris D and Littlejohns P. *Implementing clinical guidelines: a practical guide.* Abingdon: Radcliffe Medical Press, 1999.

4. Eve R *et al. Learning from FACTS.* Occasional Paper no. 97/3. Sheffield: School of Health and Related Research, 1997.

5. Ovretveit J. *Evaluating Health Interventions: An Introduction to the Evaluation of Health Treatments, Services, Policies and Organisational Interventions.* Buckingham: Open University Press, 1998.

6. Smith L and McClenahan JW. *Putting Practitioners through the Paces: Initial Findings in our evaluation of Putting Evidence into Practice.* London: King's Fund, 1997.

7. Evans D and Haines A. *Implementing Evidence-Based Changes in Health Care.* Abingdon: Radcliffe Medical Press, 2000.

8. Smith L and McClenahan JW. *Snakes and Ladders: Levers, Obstacles and Solutions to Putting Evidence Into Practice.* London: King's Fund, 1998.